Adrenal Fatigue

What Is Adrenal Fatigue Syndrome And How To Reset Your Diet And Your Life

By

Michele Gilbert

<u>Visit My Amazon Author Page</u>

Dedicated to those who choose to stretch beyond their own limits and to seek a more abundant and fulfilling life.

Your thoughts are creative.

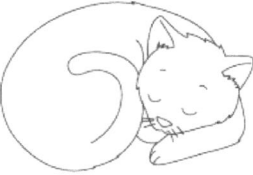

Michele Gilbert

My Free Gift To You!

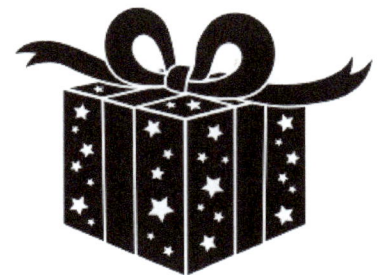

As a way of saying thank you for downloading my book, I am willing to give you access to a selected group of readers who (every week or so) receive inspiring, life-changing kindle books at deep discounts, and sometimes even absolutely free.

Wouldn't it be great to get amazing Kindle offers delivered directly to your inbox?

Wouldn't it be great to be the first to know when I'm releasing new fresh and above all sharply discounted content?

But why would I so something like this?

Why would I offer my books at such a low price and even give them away for free when they took me countless hours to produce?

Simple.... because I want to spread the word!

For a few short days Amazon allows Kindle authors to promote their newly released books by offering them deeply discounted (up to 70% price discounts and even for free. This allows us to spread the word extremely quickly allowing users to download thousands and thousands of copies in a very short period of time.

Once the timeframe has passed, these books will revert back to their normal selling price. That's why you will benefit from being the first to know when they can be downloaded for free!

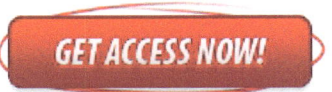

So are you ready to claim your weekly Kindle books?

You are just one click away! Follow the link below and sign up to start receiving awesome content

Thank you and Enjoy!

Table of contents

Introduction

I want to thank you and congratulate you for downloading the book, *"Adrenal Fatigue: What is Adrenal Fatigue and How to Reset Your Diet and Your Life"*

This book contains proven steps and strategies on how to identify Adrenal Fatigue, which is one of those officially "non-existing" ailments which affects thousands of people and ranges from perpetual tiredness to being totally debilitating. If you have been exhausted for months, yet cleared of any recognized illness; or are being treated for your symptoms but are not improving; this book will not only answer your questions but put you back on the road to vitality.

Adrenal Fatigue Syndrome is no respecter of age, activity, or lifestyle. It can affect students, young parents, athletes, the stressed office-worker, or the newly-retired, all unable to understand why they have suddenly run into a wall which no-one can identify. It has been misdiagnosed as depression, menopause, and a range of other fatiguing illnesses, but the recognized treatments for those won't help. Sometimes they make sufferers feel worse. If you are nearly at the end of your tether, the good news is that you've just taken the first step back.

Thanks again for downloading this book, I hope you enjoy it!

CHAPTER 1
So What Is Adrenal Fatigue

Get used to the idea right away that even if your symptoms fit like a glove, a good many people, including doctors, may tell you there is no such thing as Adrenal Fatigue. There are illnesses which share the symptoms, and you should rule those out first. The chances are, though, that you have picked this book because you've had all the tests, you've been cleared as healthy—and yet you still feel as though healthy and active is a dim and distant memory. The best thing to do next is learn as much as you can about Adrenal Fatigue. You picked the right book!

The following sections are designed to tell you the symptoms and causes of the syndrome, those likeliest to have it, the lifestyle triggers for it (and managing or changing them), the traditional and homeopathic approaches, adjusting your diet, and ways of tackling the problem generally. One thing is for sure, nothing in this book can do other than help. That's important, because some of the supplements and vitamins marketed to treat Adrenal Fatigue aren't necessarily safe, and can have the opposite effect, causing your adrenal glands more distress. Treatments can also be expensive, because medical insurance won't usually cover them.

Before you could skip straight to the next section, with the signs and symptoms, you should learn what adrenal fatigue is.

The adrenal glands are walnut-sized, situated above each kidney, and react swiftly to help you cope with difficult situations. They were originally designed to flood our systems with the boost we needed in emergencies, but the problem with modern life is that the brain is constantly reacting to what it sees as emergency situations. Stress, handled properly, is actually essential to our survival but when the button is pressed too often, triggering a body response time and again, the glands go into overdrive, or they malfunction.

There are two of them and when they are working normally they provide, in lay terms, adrenaline (the fight-or-flight hormone), noradrenaline (which reacts to fear and affects blood pressure), cortisol (which plays a role in blood sugar management and your immune system) dopamine (affecting your nervous central system) and steroids. They are essential to our wellbeing and balance. Healthy adrenal gland secretions have us feeling at our strongest and most alert at the start of the day, tapering off naturally towards the end of the day, so that we fall asleep easily, wake feeling rested, and have energy to call on.

Constant or intense stress, or respiratory infections, even a serious attack of 'flu, can affect the performance and leave you feeling tired, unwell, depressed and generally off-color. When this grat feeling can't be shaken off and becomes chronic, yet medical tests can't pick up any physical cause you have a classic Adrenal Fatigue profile. It probably isn't any consolation, but you share tha profile with millions of others.

CHAPTER 2
What Are The Signs and Symptoms of Adrenal Fatigue

It has been referred to as the 21st century stress disorder, and is often dismissed by the medical profession. In fairness to them, changes to the adrenal glands can be too slight to be picked up in medical tests, despite the impact even slight changes have to the body. To anyone suffering it, the changes may be medically slight, but they have a devastating effect on lifestyle, especially as it often affects people who eat healthily, exercise, and keep themselves in shape, yet are increasingly fatigued.

If you have several of the following symptoms, there are tests that will pick up the more alarming alternatives, listed at the end of this section. Have them done.

It is normal to experience the following occasionally. However if you can't remember when you were last free of them, you have had tests for the other ailments that share the symptoms, and your condition isn't improving despite being on medication, welcome aboard.

- Difficulty getting to sleep, despite feeling weary
- Difficulty waking up, and not feeling rested when you do
- Constant tiredness and feeling rundown
- Depression and / or nervousness
- Failing to cope with ongoing stress – feeling overwhelmed
- Trouble concentrating, thinking clearly or finishing tasks
- Slow recovery from stress or mild illness
- Craving sweet or salty snacks, or caffeine, to start or get through the day
- Body aches, headaches, and digestive disorders

What else could it be?

Unfortunately many of the symptoms are shared by several illnesses and conditions. Depression, as we all know, physically affects the body, and very often the traditional treatment is to put the patient onto anti-depressants. These won't help – in fact any chemical added to your daily intake will possibly exacerbate the condition. In middle-aged and older women it is often put down to the menopause.

Diseases which do share some or all of the symptoms are anemia, arthritis, diabetes, thyroid or heart problems, Addison's disease, tuberculosis, types of cancer, and AIDS.

No scientific proof exists to support adrenal fatigue as a true medical condition, and until there is a way of testing for it, that will remain the case. This book is for those who fall into the gray area where the serious illnesses have been **ruled out**, and yet the symptoms persist.

It is, by the way, possible to test hormone levels in saliva, but the tests have to be done several times a day, and may be both expensive and inconvenient. At time of writing, they are not covered by conventional medical aid as they are not considered conclusive. Hormone levels do change during the day. Building up a profile, to establish whether the dips and peaks are excessive, takes time, and no healthy person has a profile already on record for comparison when their health changes.

CHAPTER 3
Adrenal Fatigue What Causes It?

At its simplest, the cause is being under long-term mental, emotional, or physical stress. The death of a loved one, major surgery, severe or constant stress, even a serious attack of the 'flu, can affect the adrenal glands and the hormones that they produce. Those hormones regulate energy, the immune system, heart rate, blood pressure, muscle tone and general resilience. Any imbalance impacts on your life. Usually the glands regulate themselves eventually. When they develop fatigue, they can't regulate themselves and an acute condition becomes chronic.

You are more likely to develop the condition if you have a constantly stressful job or home life, are a shift worker, a student under prolonged pressure, or a single parent.

Abusing alcohol or drugs is another trigger, as is poor diet, although it can affect people who take care to lead a healthy lifestyle.

CHAPTER 4
Who Is Most Susceptible To Adrenal Fatigue

There is no age or stage which can't be affected. Life is stressful. School life, whether because of bullying or exam pressure, can be incredibly stressful. Marriage, parenthood, new jobs or losing jobs, repeated illnesses, are all stressful but the entire body is designed to cope with stress. In a normally functioning body hormones are released to help, we pick ourselves up and we battle on to the end of the problem. When there is no end to the problem, when the hormones are called on too often and the adrenal glands become fatigued, the condition will develop.

Statistics, because of the inaccuracy of the tests available, are difficult to judge. Low cortisol in the body *can* be measured, and if that is taken as an indicator, the percentage of people classified as potentially affected is alarmingly high – close on 60% operating at less than peak adrenal efficiency. You'll understand why doctors don't see it as a medical condition because we all cope. We just don't bounce through life.

Put it this way – depression chronically affects 1 in 5 older people. Around 25% of the population will be treated for depression in any given year.

Unofficial figures suggest as many as 80% of us will suffer chronic depression at some point. Many sufferers either don't seek treatment, or have already learned that anti-depressants don't help.

It is extremely likely that in many cases what is thought to be their mental condition causing physical symptoms could in fact turn out to be a physical cause - adrenal fatigue - causing their depression.

CHAPTER 5
Adrenal Fatigue The Effects Of Lifestyle And Nutrition

The commonest triggers are listed, and defined, below. Check the definitions; you may be surprised to find that what is perfectly normal to you is actually a known trigger. In nearly every case history there was a combination of factors which were being successfully juggled, until one final factor triggered the overload. You may have some habits here which go back *years*.

There are brief suggestions for reversing them, with more detail on an holistic approach in the next section.

Poor sleep habits – going to bed only when you feel sleepy, be that at three in the morning one day, midnight the next, and eight pm the night after, may feel right but is a poor sleep habit. So, however, is trying to force yourself to go to sleep at nine every night when you simply don't feel sleepy at nine. The *average* adult needs between six and eight hours sleep a night. Try to establish a sleep habit that fits your lifestyle, then stick to it at least five nights a week. Bodies respond very well to habit.

Poor diet- diet will be covered in more detail later but you don't need me to tell you that snacking from mid-morning to late at night, especially without eating a 'proper' meal isn't healthy!

Use of stimulants – caffeine, nicotine, prescription drugs and recreational or even energy-boost drugs take their toll.

Sudden change in lifestyle – moving to a new place, especially a distant one- promotions, demotions, retirement; even if you have been looking forward to the change, it puts new pressure on your ability to cope. Sometimes it can be a final straw

Stress at work- although it is the commonest culprit, sometimes stress at work is just the most obvious. Get everything else sorted, and you will find you can stay on top of the job, and even thrive on the challenge.

Stress at home-this doesn't relate only to abusive relationships. Illness in the family, a partner under difficult pressures, youngsters going through a turbulent age, marriage under fire, studying, training for a competitive event, even difficult neighbours, all contribute to stress at home. Sometimes you are so busy being supportive you don't even realize you, too, are being affected.

Self-induced stress – setting yourself difficult targets is, of course, challenging and interesting. That marathon you want to run, the examination you want to pass, the perfectionism you expect of yourself. You have to be in harmony with yourself before you add to your own load.

Too much exercise – if you are still tired 30 minutes after completing your exercise for the day, you are overdoing it.

Substance abuse- the commonest are alcohol and cigarettes, sleeping pills, and uppers. It is hard to tell someone on the edge that one or more of their crutches should be knocked away. They all take up more than their fair share of the body's resources to neutralize. But you know that.

Lack of fun or stress-relieving practices – when did you last play with the dog, talk a walk just for fun, enjoy yourself? Probably the very last thing you can imagine doing and yet you will never achieve balance without them

Trauma – serious illness, your own or someone close to you, or a disaster in your life, is incredibly isolating, but in fact you are never alone. Recognizing that there is help out there is a big step towards coping. There are support groups for every situation. You aren't the first, you won't be the last, and you will in time be able to help someone else who hadn't realized they weren't alone.

Depression- is sometime called the common cold of mental illness, and the signals to the adrenal glands are controlled by the brain. A mental imbalance will create a physical one – in some cases adrenal fatigue and depression are a chicken-and-egg situation, and in those cases diagnosis and treatment *will* help.

CHAPTER 6
Natural Methods Of Treating Adrenal Fatigue

First and best – sleep! The more tired you are, the more pressure you put on your fatigued glands to keep you upright and moving. More easily said than done, you will say, but try the following suggestions rather than taking sleeping pills and throwing yet more chemicals into the mix.

- Set a bedtime. Think back to when you last slept well on a regular basis. Eleven o'clock? Eleven o'clock it is. Keep to it. The occasional later night, or heading to bed earlier, should be kept to the minimum. Eventually, they won't be a problem, but establish a habit first. If you've been going to bed at nine because you're so tired, but waking at two, adjusting your sleep time will be exhausting but worth trying for a week. You should allow for eight hours of sleep, then adjust that if you find you need more, or less. Eight hours is only a suggestion; what used to work for you in the days when you slept well is a good starting point.

- Don't eat too near your bedtime, whatever time that is. Try for a minimum of two hours before you plan to turn in.

- Wind down before you go to bed, not only when you get there. Don't work, or watch something complicated on TV, or read a book with cliff-hangers, right up to bedtime. Take ten minutes to trace a peaceful memory of a park, or a beach, if you can't clear your mind without a focus.

- Sufferers tend to be tired all day, then find a late push of energy in the evening. Use it for some undemanding exercise, like a walk – not a power walk, either. Wind down. Look about you. Take a walking stick (no matter how young you are) and lop the heads off weeds. See how accurate you are at tapping the stick down on specific spots while you're walking (it's remarkably distracting). If you're up to something more strenuous, keep it moderate until you are back to health.

Sort out your diet. Bad eating habits put a strain on the whole system, which has to perform on inferior fuel. There are guidelines in the next section.

Learn to say no. You can't do everything. If you have to take on something new, then you have to lose something you were already doing. If it is work, no-one will thank you for taking on too much and missing targets. Far better to say you'd be happy to do Z, but who then will take on Y, as it isn't going to be possible to do both? It's a chance to lose your least favourite task, and a reminder to the hierarchy that you cover a whole alphabet already. If it is another task at home that can't be avoided, other tasks will have to be re-shuffled.

Learn to say no to yourself, as well. It's great to have aims and ambitions, but make them realistic. Failure is demoralizing. Pace yourself.

Take some physical time out - this is not the late-night walk, this is a physical break at some point during the day. Turn the mind off to stop sending its barrage of signals to the adrenal glands. The exercise should be moderate, or you're triggering a different series of demands. Yoga, swimming, walking the dog (borrow one if you have to), lifting weights. Even half an hour of stretching the body and resting the mind is going to make a difference. You'll sleep better, too.

If you **do smoke or drink alcohol,** at least don't combine that with anything else. If you have a drink or a cigarette, that should be *all* you do. Stop everything else. Ideally take it outside. You'll find surprisingly soon that when you have to stop everything, the breaks become naturally further and further apart. When you *do* take the breaks, they are quiet times, and that helps too.

Take a good hard look at your life – what is stressing you? Most of our chains, whether we realize it or not, we draped around ourselves. You may be the best person to do something, but unless you are alone on a desert island, you are not the only person. If you broke a leg tomorrow, who would take over?

Some chains can be dropped. Some can be handed over. Some can be lightened to essentials.

Happy hour – make a happy hour. Family. Friends. Pets. Watch a show you like on TV. Read. Be happy for an hour. It is the hardest thing on this list to do, for an adrenal fatigue sufferer, but the most beneficial.

CHAPTER 7
Adrenal Fatigue Eating Guidelines

For many adrenal fatigue sufferers, an eating plan has become a coffee kick-start, the first packet of crisps mid-morning with a fizzy drink high in caffeine, a scratch meal of a sort around noon and alternating sweet and savoury snacks with more caffeine until bedtime. However, even those who watch their diet scrupulously, and would be horrified by the thought of candy treats, can be sufferers.

So what constitutes an eating plan, and can you live with a complicated list of requirements or will you be back to your old habits in three days because they're easier?

There are hundreds of very good recipe books with simple healthy meals. Unless you get a kick from that sort of thing, avoid the complicated clever ones that have you drizzling elegant substances over food you have always avoided, which take an hour to prepare. It is far more important to set rules for yourself which are sensible, practical and fit into your lifestyle. Some foods have to go. Some have to be brought in. You are a sensible adult with a problem that is affecting your quality of life, and you want to fix it. Here are the guidelines.

As a general rule of thumb, **cut way back on over-processed foods** and get back to a natural diet. Get into that habit for life anyway, because your entire body will prefer it, not just your adrenal glands. Proteins, the good fats, vegetables, are core to your recovery diet. Fruit and carbs are okay, but in moderation while you're on a recovery diet. Regular healthy snacks keep your energy levels topped up. Don't get too hungry, and don't overeat; moderation, again. This isn't a diet to lose weight; olive oil, butter, cheese are welcome. In fact your lifestyle has probably affected your insulin levels, which directly affects your weight. Sorting out the problem could sort out any weight issues you have, too, but since you are eating in moderation, you won't be setting up other problems for the future.

Take your time about eating, even if it is only ten minutes for the snacks. Do *not* eat and work at the same time. Chew your food well, and slowly, to speed up digestion.

It is incredibly easy for a nutritionist to say cut out all sugar, caffeine and junk food, but if you're going to fall off that wagon promptly, just try to keep **everything in moderation**. You don't need ten cups of coffee a day, but one cup won't kill you. Drink a lot more filtered (rather than bottled) water and try the herbal teas.

Don't starve yourself, and don't overeat. Your healthy stomach, at rest, is the size of your fist. If you have an over-eating pattern, serve yourself a plate of food, and then put half of it back in the warmer drawer. Eat slowly, chewing well. Wait half an hour. Then you can eat the other half, but you will probably find you don't have the appetite to finish it. Not wasted: pop it in the fridge, or even freeze it. If it can be frozen, that's a snack you'll enjoy in three days.

You have to start eating **breakfast**. It is your route back to health, like it or not, because your fatigued adrenals need help kick-starting you for the day. However, the usual recommendations aren't necessarily the best for your condition. That glass of orange juice is not the best idea. The sugary cereal, ditto. Fish, cold meat, eggs, are your best breakfast friends. Multigrain toast is far better than white. If you can't face food first thing in the morning, or really don't have time, hard-boiled eggs are quick and handy for mid-morning. Eat by 10 or you'll be flagging again – the sooner after you wake up, though, the better.

If you ate early, **have a snack mid-morning**. Nuts are easy, a slice of cheese, natural yoghurt, a slice of chicken or a drumstick, sliced raw vegetables, are all good. Crisps are a no-no for now. Sorry. Stick to natural.

Don't leave it too long between meals, you're fuelling here. **Lunch** should be around noon, and a big salad with some additional protein – a tuna salad, or some chicken – is ideal. Add nuts, sunflower seeds, olive oil, make it look and taste good.

A mid-afternoon snack can include fruit; your system is fully awake by now. Whole fruit is better, because it comes complete with fiber to aid digestion.

Dinner – ideally around 6 pm, to keep up the fuel pattern – high in protein again. Fried food is not a great idea near bedtime. Bulk up with vegetables or a salad.

If you crave an **evening snack** around 8 pm, have one. I'm not the boss of you. However, keep it simple and digestible and not too sugary, otherwise you'll be jazzing yourself up for bedtime.

The essentials to remember are actually pretty simple.

- **Eat regularly**, ideally topping up at 2-3 hour intervals, while you're in recovery.

- Real food. The more processed it is, the longer a life it has, the tougher it will be on your system. Preservatives are not your friend.

- White sugar, white flour, is over-processed. Still, sugar is better than using a sweetener. If you are switching to herbal teas, try them without sugar at all. Avoid white bread and try the whole-grains instead.

- Butter is more easily digested than most margarines. Dairy generally is good, but flavour your own natural yoghurt rather than buying the pre-flavoured. Cheese that feels like rubber is not cheese!

- Raw or lightly cooked food is quick and easy, especially for those snacks.

- Cut back on fruit and push up on salads and vegetables, at least for now. Fructose makes your body work harder than you realize. No problem with a healthy digestion: tough on one in meltdown.

- Rotate your meals; it can be tempting, when you find a daily menu that is easy to put together, to eat the same foods every day. Try rather to have a three day plan. Easy to shop for, and three days between repeated meals is ideal.

- Organic food is a little more expensive but either chemical-free or at the very least dramatically less than the mass-produced stuff. The chemicals that organic farms are permitted to use are strictly monitored and are adrenal-friendly. Free-range chickens taste better and also lay better eggs. There's an old saying we all seem to have forgotten – a dollar spent on the table is a dollar saved at the doctor. Buy quality wherever possible.

Additives, once you fix your diet, shouldn't be necessary. If you are finding it difficult to eat enough of the following, you can top up with organic alternatives available across the counter:

Omega 3 fatty acids – salmon, mackerel, herring, tuna or cod liver oil capsules

Mineral sea salt rather than conventional salt

Vitamin C - citrus, strawberries, and green leafy vegetables.

Vitamin B – liver, meat, seafood, vegetables. Marmite is a yeast-based spread suitable for vegetarians which is high in Vitamin B, making it a very handy snack.

CONCLUSION
Every day, in every way, getting better and better...

You aren't on your own. It isn't a five-minute fix but in a year you will look back on this time as bad dream and will have set yourself up on a healthy lifestyle for life into the bargain. Thank yo again for downloading this book!

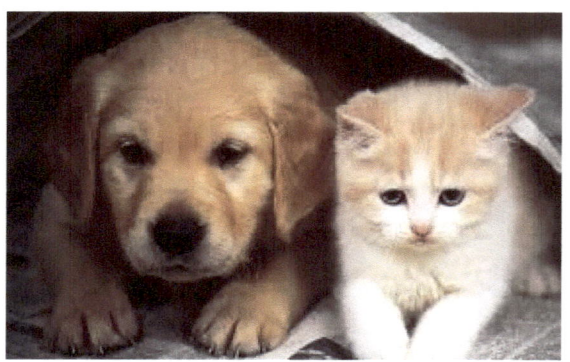

Before you go, I'd like to say thank you for purchasing my book.

I know you could have picked so many other books to read on overcoming rejection. But you took chance on me.

So A Big thanks for downloading this book and reading it all the way to completion.

Now I would like to ask a _small_ favor.

Could you please take a minute or two to leave a review for this book on Amazon?

Click here

The feedback will help me continue to publish more kindle books that will help people to get bette results in their lives.

And if you found it helpful in anyway then please let me know :-)

Preview of My New Book

What A Person's Body Language Is Really Telling You… And How You Can Use It To Your Advantage

Talk to the Hand

I don't know about you, but when I watch shows like *Lie to Me* or *Sherlock*, so often, I really, really wish that I could be that good. Heck, after I watched *The Mentalist* for the first time, I was studying everyone. I stared at footprints trying to see if I could tell whether the person walking was right handed or left handed. Not only is this super impractical for me as an actual skill, but it's super addicting. The thing is, it's all about studying people and watching them, but there's a science to it. I may not be out there catching criminals red handed for having a nervous tell, but it has helped me read situations and understand things that I previously missed.

So sure, you might not catch your arch-nemesis, but you might be able to understand things a little better with a little study of body language. And that's why I'm here. Body language is not just for detectives out there looking to catch murderers and thieves. Body language is the key to understanding the unspoken words that our body is communicating so heavily without our knowledge. Not only will this help you understand and relate to people better, but it'll make it so that you are aware of your own presence to others.

Nonverbal communication makes up the majority of our communication and most of us are clueless to the actual comprehension and understanding of it. That means that those who do not invest time in learning what to say in our nonverbal appearance are missing so much. But the truth is, we don't miss all of it. We have come to silently absorb and understand nonverbal communication, regardless of whether we know it or not. It's the art of learning to understand something we already know and to heighten our understanding and acceptance of what's being communicated to us. It's tricky, I know, but it's not impossible to understand.

What I'm going to tell you in this book is going to make sense to you and a lot of it is going to feel familiar, like you already knew that. Well, the reason for that is that you you've been picking up these silent transmissions for years, you just haven't acknowledged them or put a name to some of the habits you've already taught yourself.

So stick around and start to see if you can't agree or relate to some of the information you're going to receive. But more importantly, I want to address your homework before we start getting into the gritty, deep stuff. For instance, I want you to start watching people around you.

Observation is the birth of understanding and without a true sense of observance or a keen eye for noticing the little things, you're not going to pick up on some of these traits. When someone is talking to you, you're going to need to start watching them. Notice how they're standing, note the posture, have you looked at their eyes, what about the overall harmony of their face, and what are they doing with their hands? All of these things need to be running through your mind to really catch what is being conveyed to you. But not just watching their body, note the tones they're using and the words that they're selecting. These are all going to tell you what sort of body language comes with certain attitudes and emotions. It all ties together and it is all relevant when it comes to understanding body language. So start opening your eyes and let's have a look at what they're trying to say to you.

Are you ready?

Weapons of Mass Induction

Though Sherlock Holmes often touts his use of deductive reasoning, it is actually the opposite that we're going to focus on with you, because right now, you're a student. For those of you that do not know, inductive reasoning starts with observations that slowly build a pattern that you will then form into a hypothesis until it is proven right or wrong. If you're right, then you have a theory.

For example, Kayla touches her hair a lot when she talks to Hot Mike, but not when she's talking to anyone else. So, every time I see Kayla talking to Hot Mike and she's touching her hair, that might be a cue that she likes Hot Mike. So, until I'm proven wrong, I'm certain that I have a theory that when a woman likes a man, she'll touch her hair unconsciously.

Viola, you have just jumped from observation to theory until proven wrong. Of course, when you're Sherlock Holmes level, you'll be using the art of deductive reasoning which starts at a theory and then tested with a hypothesis and observations until you have a conclusion. I think it's time for another example to prove this one to you.

[Click Here To Read The Rest of](#)

[Body Language 101](#)

[What A Person's Body Language Is Really Telling You... And How You Can Use It To Your Advantage](#)

P.S. You'll find many more books like this and others under my name Michele Gilbert.

Don't miss them... here is a short list.

Wicca: The Ultimate Beginners Guide For Witches and Warlocks: Learn Wicca Magic

The Introvert's Advantage: The Introverts Guide To Succeeding In An Extrovert World

Stop Playing Mind Games: How To Free Yourself Of Controlling And Manipulating Relationships

Instant Charisma: A Quick And Easy Guide To Talk, Impress, And Make Anyone Like You

Chakras: Understanding The 7 Main Chakras For Beginners: The Ultimate Guide To Chakra Mindfulness, Balance and Healing

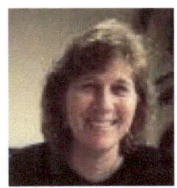

Michele Gilbert was born and raised in Brooklyn, New York. Drawn to literature and writing at a young age, she enrolled at Brooklyn College and majored in English. After graduation Michele did not begin writing immediately, instead she embarked on a career in the finance industry and spent the next thirty years on Wall Street.

Serendipity struck when she least expected it. After ending a long-term relationship, Michele found herself lost and unsure what the future held. She began to read books on grief and loss, looking for answers. Those led her to delve deeper into the Law of Attraction and its power. What resulted was remarkable. Not only had she begun to heal, she had also rekindled her former love of writing and discovered her life's purpose.

The years have taken her through many twists and turns, but she learned valuable lessons along the way. Today she publishes books-mostly self-help and metaphysical in nature-and feels compelled to share her knowledge with those facing similar experiences. Her greatest hope is to inspire others and show them ways to overcome adversity and gracefully accept life's inevitable low points.

Going forward, she plans to incorporate more teachings of self-help, finance and meditation. Regular meditation is very beneficial to her progress as she forges a new life. Morning rituals and positive incantations are other practices Michele embraces; they are very restorative in daily life.

As an avid hiker, Michele and fellow club members often hike the picturesque Jersey Pine Barrens. She is a history buff, voracious reader, baseball fanatic and a foodie. She also proudly supports Trout Unlimited-a national non-profit organization dedicated to conserving, protecting and restoring North America's Coldwater fisheries and their watersheds.

Michele currently resides forty minutes from Atlantic City and the Jersey Shore. She makes her home with a Blue Russian rescue cat named Jersey, though she isn't exactly sure who rescued who.

Michele really enjoys publishing books that can make a difference in people's lives. If you have any suggestions or would like to have a specific topic covered in a future book, please send an email to michelegilbertbooks@gmail.com and we will get back to you.

Thanks for reading!

www.ingramcontent.com/pod-product-compliance
Lightning Source LLC
Chambersburg PA
CBHW050930290526
45792CB00002B/957